Unlocking the Cholesterol Puzzle: Your Essential Guide to Understanding the 'Good' and 'Bad' of Cholesterol!

Flora S. Trevino

INTRODUCTION

"Did you know that in the intricate symphony of your body's health, there's a 'good' and 'bad' player called Cholcholestrol? Discover the key to mastering this symphony for a healthier, harmonious life!"

Cholesterol is like the backstage manager of your body's health – it orchestrates the performance of your organs and systems. Within this complex symphony, there are key players: LDL (low-density lipoprotein) and HDL (high-density lipoprotein), often tagged as the 'bad' and 'good' cholesterol. Understanding their roles is pivotal in mastering your body's health.

Cholesterol 101

Cholesterol, often misunderstood as a dietary foe, is a fundamental component of cell membranes and a precursor for steroid hormones and bile acids. It's synthesized in the liver and obtained through diet, playing a crucial role in various bodily functions.

The Dance of LDL and HDL

LDL, known as the 'bad' cholesterol, ferries cholesterol from the liver to cells but can accumulate in artery walls, leading to plaques and cardiovascular issues. On the other hand, HDL, the 'good' cholesterol, scavenges excess cholesterol from cells and transports it back to the liver for excretion, reducing the risk of artery blockages.

The Heart-Cholesterol Connections

High LDL levels and low HDL levels are associated with an increased risk of heart disease, strokes, and other cardiovascular complications. Atherosclerosis, the buildup of plaques in arteries, is primarily linked to high LDL cholesterol.

Measuring the Cholesterol Score

Lipid profile tests provide insights into cholesterol levels. Total cholesterol, LDL, HDL, and triglycerides are measured, guiding health professionals in assessing an individual's cardiovascular risk.

Managing Cholesterol Naturally

Dietary modifications, such as reducing saturated and trans fats while embracing healthier fats like omega-3 fatty acids, can positively influence cholesterol levels. Incorporating soluble fiber, found in fruits, vegetables, and whole grains, aids in lowering LDL cholesterol.

Regular physical activity, especially aerobic exercises, boosts HDL levels and helps control weight, indirectly impacting cholesterol levels.

Beyond Lifestyle: Medications and Interventions

In many instances, , certain behavioral changes might not be sufficient. Medications like statins, which inhibit cholesterol production in the liver, are prescribed to manage high cholesterol. Other medications and interventions exist for specific conditions or genetic predispositions affecting cholesterol.

Navigating Your Cholesterol Journey

Understanding the nuances of cholesterol management is empowering. Overcoming challenges, maintaining consistency in lifestyle changes, and staying motivated are crucial for long-term success in managing cholesterol levels.

Conclusion:

Mastering cholesterol isn't about eliminating it but striking a balance. It's about embracing the 'good' and managing the 'bad' to compose a symphony of health.

Chapter one :

Cholesterol Unveiled

Cholesterol, often portrayed as a dietary villain, is far more than its infamous reputation suggests. Imagine cholesterol as the building blocks of your body's cellular framework, an unsung hero facilitating essential bodily functions. Understanding its intricate role unveils a narrative crucial to your overall health.

At its core, cholesterol is a waxy, fat-like substance coursing through your bloodstream and embedded within every cell membrane. Contrary to common belief, it's not all "bad." In fact, it's indispensable, serving as a foundation for vital processes within your body.

One of cholesterol's primary roles is the construction and maintenance of cell membranes. Without these membranes, cells wouldn't maintain their structural integrity or function optimally. Cholesterol acts as the stabilizing agent, preventing excessive fluidity or rigidity in cell membranes, thus ensuring proper cellular function.

Additionally, this multifaceted substance plays a pivotal role in hormone production. Cholesterol is a precursor for the synthesis of steroid hormones, including cortisol, estrogen, and testosterone. These hormones regulate various bodily functions, such as metabolism, stress response, reproductive health, and more.

But wait, there's more to this complex narrative! Cholesterol takes center stage in aiding digestion by supporting the production of bile acids. These acids facilitate the breakdown of dietary fats, allowing their absorption in the intestines. This critical process ensures proper nutrient uptake and utilization throughout the body.

Cholesterol's journey within the body involves transportation through lipoproteins, specifically LDL (low-density lipoprotein), HDL (high-density lipoprotein), and VLDL (very-low-density lipoprotein). These carriers ensure cholesterol reaches its designated destinations, contributing to various bodily functions while maintaining a delicate balance.

While cholesterol is indeed indispensable, an imbalance in its levels can spell trouble. High levels of LDL cholesterol, often termed 'bad' cholesterol, can lead to the buildup of plaques in artery walls, increasing the risk of heart disease and stroke. Conversely, elevated levels of HDL cholesterol, the 'good' counterpart, can reduce these risks by transporting excess cholesterol away from arteries to the liver for disposal.

In essence, cholesterol, far from being a simple dietary foe, is a nuanced protagonist in your body's symphony. Understanding its multifaceted nature unveils a narrative essential to your overall health, shedding light on the intricate interplay of cholesterol's roles and the delicate balance required for optimal well-being.

Detailing the composition and role of cholesterol in the body.

Cholesterol, often misconstrued as a dietary enemy, is an indispensable molecule crucial for various bodily functions. Its composition, a waxy, fat-like substance, renders it a fundamental building block within the intricate framework of the human body.

Composition of Cholesterol:

Chemically, cholesterol belongs to the lipid family, characterized by its inability to dissolve in water. Structurally, it comprises four interconnected hydrocarbon rings, distinguishing it from other lipids. This unique arrangement allows cholesterol to integrate seamlessly into cell membranes, ensuring their stability and fluidity.

Cholesterol's Role in the Body:

Cell Membrane Integrity:

Cholesterol plays a pivotal role in constructing and maintaining cell membranes. Within these membranes, cholesterol's presence regulates their fluidity, preventing excessive rigidity or fluidity. This regulation is vital for cellular function, ensuring the proper passage of nutrients and waste products across the cell.

Hormone Production:

As a precursor molecule, cholesterol serves as the foundation for synthesizing steroid hormones. These hormones, including cortisol, aldosterone, estrogen, and testosterone, play diverse roles in regulating metabolism, stress responses, electrolyte balance, reproductive functions, and more.

Bile Acid Synthesis:

Cholesterol contributes significantly to the creation of bile acids within the liver. These acids are crucial for the breakdown and absorption of dietary fats in the intestines. Bile acids emulsify fats, enabling their digestion and absorption, ensuring proper nutrient utilization in the body.

Vitamin D Synthesis:

Cholesterol serves as a precursor for the synthesis of vitamin D, a vital nutrient responsible for regulating calcium and phosphorus absorption in the intestines. Adequate vitamin D levels are essential for maintaining bone health and supporting immune function.

Transportation of Cholesterol:

Cholesterol travels through the bloodstream packaged within lipoproteins, which act as carrier vehicles. LDL (low-density lipoprotein) transports cholesterol from the liver to various tissues throughout the body. Excessive LDL cholesterol can contribute to the formation of arterial plaques, increasing the risk of cardiovascular diseases.

On the contrary, HDL (high-density lipoprotein) collects excess cholesterol from tissues and arteries, transporting it back to the liver for disposal or recycling.

Conclusion:

Cholesterol, far from being a mere dietary concern, is an integral component essential for the proper functioning of the body. Its multifaceted roles, from cell membrane integrity to hormone production and nutrient absorption, underscore its significance. Understanding cholesterol's composition and pivotal functions elucidates its nuanced role within the complex orchestra of human health.

Illustrating cholesterol's multifaceted functions beyond its infamous reputation.

Cholesterol, often vilified for its association with heart disease, possesses a myriad of essential functions that extend far beyond its notorious reputation. Beyond being a mere lipid, cholesterol serves as an indispensable protagonist in maintaining overall health and vitality.

1. Cellular Architecture:

Cholesterol assumes the role of a structural architect within cell membranes. Its presence ensures the membranes' integrity and functionality by regulating fluidity. This critical function allows cells to communicate effectively, facilitating the exchange of nutrients and waste products.

2. Hormone Synthesis:

As a precursor to steroid hormones, cholesterol anchors the production of vital hormones like cortisol, aldosterone, estrogen, and testosterone. These hormones regulate various bodily functions, including stress responses, electrolyte balance, reproductive health, and metabolism.

3. Bile Production and Digestion:

Cholesterol contributes to bile acid synthesis in the liver. Bile acids, synthesized from cholesterol, play a pivotal role in emulsifying fats during digestion. This process enhances fat breakdown and facilitates the absorption of fat-soluble nutrients, such as vitamins A, D, E, and K.

4. Vitamin D Synthesis:

Cholesterol acts as a precursor in the synthesis of vitamin D, an essential nutrient for bone health and immune system function.

Sunlight triggers the conversion of cholesterol in the skin to vitamin D, highlighting cholesterol's indirect role in maintaining overall health.

5. Cell Signaling and Regulation:

Cholesterol participates in cell signaling pathways, contributing to the regulation of gene expression and cellular processes. It influences various signaling molecules, impacting cell growth, differentiation, and development.

6. Myelin Sheath Formation:

Cholesterol contributes to the formation of myelin, a protective sheath around nerve fibers essential for efficient nerve signal transmission. This role underscores its significance in maintaining proper neurological function.

7. **Antioxidant Properties:**

Studies suggest that cholesterol may possess antioxidant properties, aiding in neutralizing harmful free radicals and reducing oxidative stress within the body.

Understanding cholesterol's multifaceted functions illuminates its indispensable role in the body's orchestra of life. Beyond its often-criticized impact on heart health, cholesterol plays a pivotal part in diverse physiological processes that sustain overall well-being and vitality. Embracing this nuanced perspective shifts the narrative from mere 'bad cholesterol' to a compound orchestrating essential bodily functions.

Chapter two:

Decoding the 'Good' and 'Bad' Cholesterol**

Deciphering the distinction between 'good' and 'bad' cholesterol unveils a fundamental narrative in understanding how cholesterol impacts our health. These two entities, LDL (low-density lipoprotein) and HDL (high-density lipoprotein), each play pivotal yet distinct roles in the intricate dance of cholesterol within our bodies.

1. LDL Cholesterol: The 'Bad' Player.

LDL cholesterol, often labeled as the 'bad' cholesterol, serves as a carrier, shuttling cholesterol from the liver to various tissues throughout the body. While this function is crucial for providing cells with cholesterol for essential functions, excessive LDL levels can lead to trouble.

The problem arises when LDL particles accumulate in the walls of arteries, initiating a cascade of events leading to atherosclerosis. This buildup forms plaques that narrow arteries, impeding blood flow and potentially causing cardiovascular issues like heart attacks and strokes.

Managing LDL levels is vital; reducing its concentration can mitigate the risk of plaque formation, thus lowering the likelihood of heart disease.

2. HDL Cholesterol: The 'Good' Protector.

HDL cholesterol, in contrast, emerges as the 'good' cholesterol due to its role in safeguarding cardiovascular health. HDL acts as a scavenger, collecting excess cholesterol from tissues and arteries, and transporting it back to the liver for disposal or recycling.

Its function is akin to a cleanup crew, clearing away excess cholesterol that could potentially contribute to arterial plaque formation. Higher levels of HDL are associated with a reduced risk of heart disease, emphasizing its protective nature.

Increasing HDL levels through lifestyle modifications, such as exercise and a healthy diet, can potentially lower the risk of heart disease.

Understanding the duality of LDL and HDL cholesterol provides a crucial perspective in managing cholesterol levels. Balancing these two entities is pivotal; reducing 'bad' LDL cholesterol while bolstering 'good' HDL cholesterol can significantly impact cardiovascular health. This knowledge empowers individuals to take proactive steps in maintaining a harmonious balance between these cholesterol players for overall well-being.

Explaining LDL, HDL, and VLDL cholesterol.

Certainly! Understanding the nuances of LDL (low-density lipoprotein), HDL (high-density lipoprotein), and VLDL (very-low-density lipoprotein) cholesterol sheds light on their distinct roles and contributions to overall health.

1. **LDL Cholesterol:**

LDL cholesterol, often dubbed as the 'bad' cholesterol, primarily functions as a carrier of cholesterol throughout the body. It transports cholesterol from the liver, where it's synthesized, to various tissues and cells that require it for essential functions.

However, the trouble arises when there's an excess of LDL in the bloodstream. High levels of LDL cholesterol can lead to a buildup of cholesterol in the arterial walls, forming plaques. These plaques can narrow the arteries, impeding blood flow and increasing the risk of atherosclerosis, heart attacks, and strokes.

2. HDL Cholesterol:

HDL cholesterol, often referred to as the 'good' cholesterol, acts as a protector of cardiovascular health. Its primary role involves scavenging excess cholesterol from tissues and arteries, transporting it back to the liver for disposal or recycling.

Unlike LDL, HDL works to prevent plaque formation by clearing away excess cholesterol, thus reducing the risk of arterial blockages.

3. VLDL Cholesterol:

VLDL cholesterol, classified as very-low-density lipoprotein, primarily carries triglycerides, a type of fat, synthesized in the liver. These triglycerides are circulated throughout the body to provide energy to various tissues.

As VLDL particles release triglycerides, they transform into smaller LDL particles. Elevated levels of VLDL cholesterol are often linked to increased cardiovascular risk, similar to high LDL levels.

Each type of cholesterol plays a distinctive role in the body's lipid transport system. While LDL and VLDL are associated with potential risks when present in high levels, HDL serves a protective function. Balancing these cholesterol types through lifestyle modifications, dietary choices, and, if necessary, medical interventions can significantly impact cardiovascular health and reduce the risk of heart-related complications.

Discussing how each type impacts health and why balance is crucial.

Certainly! Each type of cholesterol—LDL (low-density lipoprotein), HDL (high-density lipoprotein), and VLDL (very-low-density lipoprotein)—exerts specific effects on health, emphasizing the critical need for a balanced cholesterol profile to maintain overall well-being.

1.LDL Cholesterol Impact:

Negative Impact: Elevated LDL levels pose a significant risk to cardiovascular health. Excess LDL cholesterol can accumulate in the arterial walls, leading to the formation of plaques. These plaques narrow the arteries, obstructing blood flow and increasing the likelihood of atherosclerosis, heart attacks, and strokes.

Importance of Balance: Keeping LDL cholesterol within optimal ranges is crucial to mitigate the risk of plaque formation and reduce the incidence of cardiovascular diseases. Managing LDL levels through dietary modifications, exercise, and medication, if necessary, is essential for maintaining cardiovascular health.

2. HDL Cholesterol Impact:

Positive Impact: Higher levels of HDL cholesterol have a protective effect on cardiovascular health. HDL acts as a scavenger, removing excess cholesterol from tissues and arteries, transporting it back to the liver for disposal or recycling.

Importance of Balance: Increasing HDL levels is associated with a reduced risk of heart disease. Balancing cholesterol levels by elevating HDL through regular exercise, healthy dietary choices, and avoiding smoking is crucial for maintaining cardiovascular health.

3. **VLDL Cholesterol Impact:**

Negative Impact: Elevated VLDL cholesterol levels are associated with increased cardiovascular risk, similar to high LDL levels. VLDL primarily carries triglycerides synthesized in the liver, and when these triglycerides are released, VLDL particles transform into smaller LDL particles.

Importance of Balance: Maintaining optimal VLDL levels, along with managing LDL and HDL cholesterol, is vital for overall cardiovascular health. Lifestyle changes, including dietary adjustments and physical activity, can positively impact VLDL levels. Why Balance is Crucial:

Achieving a balanced cholesterol profile is essential for maintaining optimal health and reducing the risk of cardiovascular diseases. Striking a balance between LDL, HDL, and VLDL cholesterol ensures proper lipid metabolism, prevents plaque formation, and supports healthy cardiovascular function.

Balanced cholesterol levels can be attained through lifestyle modifications, including a heart-healthy diet rich in fruits, vegetables, whole grains, lean proteins, and healthy fats. Regular physical activity, maintaining a healthy weight, and avoiding smoking are also pivotal in achieving and sustaining a balanced cholesterol profile.

Regular monitoring of cholesterol levels through lipid profile tests, coupled with healthcare provider guidance, allows individuals to assess their cardiovascular risk and take proactive steps to maintain a

balanced cholesterol profile for long-term health benefits.

CHapter three:

The Link Between Cholesterol and Health

The relationship between cholesterol and health is intricate, influencing various aspects of overall well-being, particularly cardiovascular health.

1. Atherosclerosis and Heart Health:

Elevated levels of LDL cholesterol play a significant role in the development of atherosclerosis, a condition characterized by the buildup of plaques in arterial walls. These plaques narrow the arteries, restricting blood flow and increasing the risk of heart disease, heart attacks, and strokes.

Lowering LDL cholesterol levels is crucial in mitigating the risk of atherosclerosis, emphasizing the need for managing cholesterol for optimal heart health.

2. Peripheral Artery Disease (PAD):

High cholesterol levels can contribute to peripheral artery disease, a condition where narrowed arteries in the legs reduce blood flow, leading to pain, numbness, or weakness in the lower extremities.

Lowering LDL cholesterol levels can alleviate the risk of PAD, highlighting cholesterol's impact on peripheral vascular health.

3. Cholesterol and Blood Pressure:

Elevated cholesterol levels, especially LDL cholesterol, can contribute to high blood pressure, further increasing the risk of cardiovascular diseases.

Managing cholesterol levels is not only vital for reducing heart disease risk but also in regulating blood pressure, promoting overall cardiovascular health.

4. **Stroke Risk:**

High levels of LDL cholesterol can contribute to the formation of blood clots or plaques in cerebral arteries, increasing the risk of stroke, which occurs when blood flow to the brain is disrupted.

Controlling cholesterol levels is essential in reducing the risk of stroke and maintaining cerebrovascular health.

Understanding the correlation between cholesterol and health underscores the importance of managing cholesterol levels for overall well-being. Lowering LDL cholesterol, while elevating HDL levels through lifestyle modifications, dietary changes, physical activity, and, if necessary, medication, is pivotal in reducing the risk of cardiovascular diseases and maintaining a healthy cardiovascular system.

Regular monitoring of cholesterol levels, coupled with adopting heart-healthy habits, empowers individuals to take proactive steps in safeguarding their cardiovascular health and reducing the incidence of cholesterol-related complications.

Unpacking the relationship between cholesterol levels and cardiovascular health.

The relationship between cholesterol levels and cardiovascular health is intricate and pivotal in determining an individual's risk of heart disease, stroke, and other cardiovascular complications.

1.LDL Cholesterol and Cardiovascular Risk:

Elevated levels of LDL (low-density lipoprotein) cholesterol significantly contribute to the development of atherosclerosis. Excess LDL cholesterol can deposit in the arterial walls, forming plaques that narrow arteries, impeding blood flow. This condition raises the risk of coronary artery disease, heart attacks, and strokes.

Lowering LDL cholesterol levels is crucial in reducing the risk of atherosclerosis and its associated cardiovascular complications.

2. HDL Cholesterol's Protective Role:

HDL (high-density lipoprotein) cholesterol plays a protective role in cardiovascular health. Higher levels of HDL are associated with a reduced risk of heart disease due to its function in scavenging excess cholesterol from tissues and arteries, transporting it back to the liver for disposal or recycling.

Increasing HDL levels through lifestyle modifications can contribute to a healthier lipid profile and reduce cardiovascular risk.

3. Triglycerides and VLDL Cholesterol:

Elevated levels of triglycerides, carried by VLDL (very-low-density lipoprotein) cholesterol, are also associated with an increased risk of cardiovascular diseases. High triglyceride levels can contribute to atherosclerosis and other cardiovascular complications.

Managing triglycerides and VLDL cholesterol levels, along with LDL and HDL, is essential in reducing overall cardiovascular risk.

4. Total Cholesterol and Cardiovascular Risk Assessment:

While LDL cholesterol is often the primary focus due to its association with atherosclerosis, evaluating total cholesterol levels, including LDL, HDL, and triglycerides, provides a more comprehensive picture of an individual's cardiovascular risk.

5. Impact of Cholesterol-Lowering Interventions:

Managing cholesterol levels through lifestyle changes, such as adopting a heart-healthy diet, regular exercise, maintaining a healthy weight, and, if necessary, medication like statins, can significantly reduce cardiovascular risk.

Understanding the relationship between cholesterol levels and cardiovascular health underscores the importance of maintaining a balanced lipid profile. Monitoring cholesterol levels regularly, adopting heart-healthy habits, and seeking medical guidance to manage cholesterol effectively are crucial steps in preventing or mitigating the risk of cardiovascular diseases. Achieving a balanced cholesterol profile plays a vital role in preserving cardiovascular health and reducing the incidence of heart-related complications.

Highlighting other health risks associated with high cholesterol.

In addition to its well-known impact on cardiovascular health, high cholesterol levels can contribute to various other health risks, emphasizing the importance of managing cholesterol for overall well-being.

1. Risk of Peripheral Artery Disease (PAD):

Elevated cholesterol levels, particularly high LDL cholesterol, can lead to the development of peripheral artery disease. This condition involves the narrowing of arteries in the legs, reducing blood flow to the extremities. PAD can manifest as leg pain, numbness, or weakness, impacting mobility and overall quality of life.

2. **Increased Risk of Stroke:**

High cholesterol levels, especially elevated LDL cholesterol, can contribute to the formation of blood clots or plaques in the cerebral arteries. These blockages or disruptions in blood flow to the brain increase the risk of stroke, a serious condition that can result in lasting neurological impairment or even death.

3. **Xanthomas and Xanthelasma:**

Excessive cholesterol levels in the blood can lead to the formation of xanthomas and xanthelasma, visible deposits of cholesterol under the skin. These can appear as yellowish bumps or patches, often around the eyelids, indicating high cholesterol levels and potentially underlying health concerns.

4. Gallstones Formation:

High cholesterol levels can contribute to the formation of gallstones in the gallbladder. Gallstones are hardened deposits that develop from cholesterol and other substances, leading to abdominal pain, nausea, and digestive issues.

5. Impact on Metabolic Syndrome:

Elevated cholesterol levels are often associated with metabolic syndrome, a cluster of conditions that include high blood pressure, insulin resistance, excess abdominal fat, and abnormal cholesterol levels. Metabolic syndrome increases the risk of heart disease, stroke, and type 2 diabetes.

6. Potential Impact on Liver Health:

Excessive cholesterol levels may impact liver health, contributing to non-alcoholic fatty liver disease (NAFLD). NAFLD involves the accumulation of fat in the liver and can progress to more severe liver conditions, such as non-alcoholic steatohepatitis (NASH) and liver fibrosis.

Managing cholesterol levels through lifestyle modifications, dietary changes, regular exercise, and, if necessary, medication can help mitigate these additional health risks associated with high cholesterol. Monitoring cholesterol levels and addressing lifestyle factors are crucial in reducing the incidence of these health complications and preserving overall health and well-being.

Chapter Four

Measuring and Understanding Cholesterol Levels

Measuring and understanding cholesterol levels involves assessing various components through a lipid profile test. This test provides valuable insights into an individual's cholesterol status, guiding healthcare professionals in evaluating cardiovascular risk.

1. **Total Cholesterol:**

Total cholesterol measures the sum of different cholesterol types present in the bloodstream, including LDL, HDL, and a fraction of VLDL. Optimal total cholesterol levels vary based on individual health factors but generally aim for lower levels of LDL and higher levels of HDL.

2.LDL Cholesterol:

LDL cholesterol, often termed 'bad' cholesterol, requires careful monitoring. Elevated LDL levels increase the risk of plaque formation in arteries, contributing to atherosclerosis and cardiovascular diseases. Ideal LDL cholesterol levels typically vary based on an individual's risk factors but generally aim for lower values to reduce cardiovascular risk.

3. HDL Cholesterol:

HDL cholesterol, referred to as 'good' cholesterol, plays a protective role by removing excess cholesterol from arteries and transporting it back to the liver for disposal. Optimal HDL levels vary but typically aim for higher values to support cardiovascular health.

4. **Triglycerides:**

Triglycerides, a type of fat in the blood, are measured alongside cholesterol levels. Elevated triglyceride levels, often associated with VLDL cholesterol, can increase cardiovascular risk. Lowering triglyceride levels through lifestyle changes is crucial for overall heart health.

5. **Understanding the Ratios:**

Ratios like the LDL/HDL ratio and total cholesterol/HDL ratio provide additional insights into cardiovascular risk. Lower ratios are generally indicative of a lower risk of heart disease.

Interpreting cholesterol levels involves considering various factors such as age, sex, family history, and other health conditions. Healthcare professionals use these lipid profile results to assess an individual's cardiovascular risk and develop personalized strategies for cholesterol management.

Regular monitoring of cholesterol levels, typically recommended every few years or more frequently based on risk factors, allows individuals to track changes and adjust lifestyle habits or treatment plans accordingly.

Understanding the significance of each cholesterol component and its implications on cardiovascular health empowers individuals to actively engage in managing their cholesterol levels for optimal heart health.

Explaining lipid profile tests and their significance in determining cholesterol levels.

A lipid profile test is a blood test that measures various components related to cholesterol and fats in the bloodstream. It provides critical information about an individual's cholesterol levels and helps assess their risk of developing cardiovascular diseases.

Here's an overview of the components measured in a lipid profile test and their significance:

1. **Total Cholesterol:**

Total cholesterol measures the overall amount of cholesterol in the blood, encompassing LDL, HDL, and a portion of VLDL cholesterol. It serves as a baseline marker for evaluating cardiovascular risk.

2. **Low-Density Lipoprotein (LDL) Cholesterol:**

LDL cholesterol is often referred to as 'bad' cholesterol. It transports cholesterol from the liver to various tissues in the body. Elevated LDL levels are associated with an increased risk of atherosclerosis and heart disease.

3. High-**Density Lipoprotein (HDL) Cholesterol:**

HDL cholesterol is known as 'good' cholesterol. It functions by removing excess cholesterol from the bloodstream and arterial walls, transporting it back to the liver for disposal.

4.Triglycerides:

It is found in the blood. Elevated triglyceride levels, especially when accompanied by high LDL cholesterol, can increase the risk of heart disease and contribute to atherosclerosis.

Significance of Lipid Profile Tests:

Cardiovascular Risk Assessment:
Lipid profile tests provide valuable information for evaluating an individual's risk of developing heart disease, strokes, and other cardiovascular conditions. Elevated LDL and total cholesterol, along with low HDL and high triglycerides, can indicate an increased risk.

Treatment Guidance: Results from lipid profile tests guide healthcare professionals in determining appropriate treatment strategies. Lifestyle modifications, dietary changes, exercise, and medication may be recommended based on the test results and an individual's risk factors.

Monitoring Progress: Regular lipid profile tests help monitor the effectiveness of interventions aimed at managing cholesterol levels. They allow for adjustments in treatment plans or lifestyle modifications based on changes in cholesterol levels over time.

Understanding the significance of each component measured in a lipid profile test aids in assessing an individual's cardiovascular risk and guides healthcare professionals in developing personalized strategies to manage cholesterol levels for optimal heart health.

Outlining optimal ranges for different cholesterol components.

Here are the generally recommended optimal ranges for different cholesterol components:

1. Total Cholesterol:

Optimal Range: Less than 200 milligrams per deciliter (mg/dL).

- Borderline High: 200-239 mg/dL.

- High: 240 mg/dL and above.

2. Low-Density Lipoprotein (LDL) Cholesterol:

- Optimal Range: Less than 100 mg/dL (for individuals with a higher risk of heart disease, the target may be lower, around 70 mg/dL).

- Borderline High: 130-159 mg/dL.

- High: 160 mg/dL and above.

3. High-Density Lipoprotein (HDL) Cholesterol:

- Optimal Range: 60 mg/dL or higher.

- Acceptable Range: 40-59 mg/dL (for men).

- Acceptable Range: 50-59 mg/dL (for women).

4. Triglycerides:

- Optimal Range: Less than 150 mg/dL.

- Borderline High: 150-199 mg/dL.

- High: 200-499 mg/dL.

- Very High: 500 mg/dL and above.

It's important to note that these ranges can vary slightly depending on individual health factors, age, presence of other health conditions, and specific risk profiles. Healthcare professionals may set individualized targets based on an individual's overall health and cardiovascular risk.

Achieving and maintaining cholesterol levels within these optimal ranges, especially by keeping LDL cholesterol low and HDL cholesterol high, contributes significantly to reducing the risk of heart disease, strokes, and other cardiovascular complications. Regular monitoring and discussions with healthcare providers help in assessing and managing cholesterol levels for optimal heart health.

Chapter Five

Managing Cholesterol Naturally

Managing cholesterol naturally involves adopting healthy lifestyle habits that can positively impact cholesterol levels. Here are some effective strategies:

1. Healthy Diet:

- Embrace a Plant-Based Diet: Include plenty of fruits, vegetables, whole grains, legumes, nuts, and seeds. These foods are rich in fiber, antioxidants, and plant sterols that can help lower LDL cholesterol.

- Omega-3 Fatty Acids: Incorporate sources of omega-3s, such as fatty fish (like salmon, mackerel, or sardines), flaxseeds, chia seeds, and walnuts, which can help raise HDL cholesterol.

- Limit Added Sugars and Refined Carbs: Reduce intake of sugary beverages, sweets, and refined carbohydrates as they can raise triglyceride levels.

2. Regular Physical Activity:

- Activities like brisk walking, jogging, cycling, or swimming can help raise HDL cholesterol and lower LDL cholesterol and triglycerides.

3. Maintain a Healthy Weight:

- Losing excess weight, especially around the midsection, can positively impact cholesterol levels. A healthy weight reduces LDL cholesterol and triglycerides while increasing HDL cholesterol.

4. Quit Smoking:

- Smoking can lower HDL cholesterol and damage blood vessels, increasing the risk of heart disease. Quitting smoking improves overall cardiovascular health.

5. Limit Alcohol Intake:

- Moderation is key. Excessive alcohol consumption can increase triglyceride levels. Men should limit alcohol to no more than two drinks per day, and women to one drink per day.

6. Manage Stress:

- Chronic stress can impact cholesterol levels. Practice stress-relieving activities like yoga, meditation, deep breathing exercises, or hobbies to manage stress effectively.

7. Get Adequate Sleep:

- Lack of sleep can affect cholesterol metabolism. Aim for 7-9 hours of quality sleep per night to support overall health, including cholesterol levels.

8. Consider Functional Foods or Supplements:

- Some foods or supplements, like oatmeal, psyllium husk, garlic, green tea, or plant sterol-enriched foods, may have cholesterol-lowering properties.

Adopting these lifestyle changes not only helps manage cholesterol levels naturally but also contributes to overall cardiovascular health. It's essential to consult a healthcare provider before making significant dietary or lifestyle changes, especially if there are existing health conditions or medications being taken. Regular monitoring and guidance from healthcare professionals are crucial in managing cholesterol effectively.

Providing dietary recommendations to control cholesterol levels.

Certainly! Here are dietary recommendations aimed at controlling cholesterol levels:

1. **Increase Fiber Intake:**

- Soluble Fiber: Foods rich in soluble fiber, such as oats, barley, legumes (beans, lentils), fruits (apples, oranges, berries), and vegetables (brussels sprouts, carrots), can help lower LDL cholesterol by reducing its absorption in the bloodstream.

2. Choose Healthier Fats:

- Monounsaturated and Polyunsaturated Fats: Sources include olive oil, avocados, nuts (almonds, walnuts, pistachios), seeds (flaxseeds, chia seeds), and fatty fish (salmon, mackerel, sardines). These fats can improve cholesterol levels, especially by increasing HDL cholesterol.

- Omega-3 Fatty Acids: Incorporate fatty fish, flaxseeds, chia seeds, and walnuts, which contain omega-3s beneficial for heart health.

3. Limit Saturated and Trans Fats:

- Reduce Red Meat and Full-Fat Dairy: Limit intake of fatty cuts of meat and full-fat dairy products as they contain saturated fats that can raise LDL cholesterol levels.

- Avoid Trans Fats: Minimize consumption of processed foods, fast food, and commercially baked goods containing trans fats, as they can increase LDL cholesterol and lower HDL cholesterol.

4. **Consume Plant Sterols and Stanols:**

- Fortified Foods: Incorporate foods enriched with plant sterols and stanols, like certain margarines, orange juice, or yogurt, which can help lower LDL cholesterol.

5. **Eat More Fish:**

- Fatty Fish: Include fish rich in omega-3 fatty acids, like salmon, mackerel, trout, and sardines, at least twice a week. These omega-3s can help improve cholesterol levels.

6. **Increase Fruit and Vegetable Intake:**

- Colorful Produce: Consume a variety of fruits and vegetables rich in antioxidants, vitamins, and minerals. These can help manage cholesterol levels and support overall heart health.

7. Limit Added Sugars and Refined Carbohydrates:

- Cut Down on Sweets and Processed Foods: Reducing intake of sugary beverages, sweets, and refined carbohydrates helps control triglyceride levels, which impact overall cholesterol health.

8. Portion Control and Balanced Meals:

- Control Portions: Pay attention to portion sizes to manage overall calorie intake and maintain a healthy weight.

- Balanced Meals: Focus on balanced meals with a mix of lean proteins, whole grains, healthy fats, and plenty of fruits and vegetables to promote overall heart health.

9. Read Food Labels:

- Be Mindful of Labels: Check food labels for hidden sources of saturated fats, trans fats, and added sugars. Choose products with lower amounts of these components.

Adopting a heart-healthy diet focused on whole, nutrient-dense foods and limiting processed and unhealthy fats can significantly impact cholesterol levels and overall cardiovascular health. It's crucial to combine dietary changes with regular physical activity and a healthy lifestyle for optimal cholesterol management. Consulting a healthcare professional or a registered dietitian can provide personalized guidance for managing cholesterol through diet effectively.

Emphasizing the importance of exercise, stress management, and lifestyle changes.

Absolutely, lifestyle modifications beyond diet play a crucial role in managing cholesterol levels and promoting overall cardiovascular health. Here's why exercise, stress management, and lifestyle changes are pivotal:

1. **Regular Exercise:**

- Improves Lipid Profile: Engaging in regular physical activity, such as aerobic exercises (walking, running, cycling, swimming), can increase HDL cholesterol levels and lower LDL cholesterol and triglycerides.

- Enhances Heart Health: Exercise supports overall cardiovascular health by strengthening the heart muscle, improving blood circulation, and reducing the risk of heart disease and stroke.

- Aids Weight Management: Physical activity assists in maintaining a healthy weight, which positively impacts cholesterol levels.

2. **Stress Management:**

- Stress and Cholesterol: Chronic stress can contribute to higher cholesterol levels. Implementing stress management techniques, such as meditation, yoga, deep breathing exercises, or mindfulness, helps lower stress hormones that can affect cholesterol.

- Improves Overall Health: Managing stress not only benefits cholesterol levels but also supports mental health, overall well-being, and heart health.

3. **Lifestyle Changes:**

- Quitting Smoking: Smoking can lower HDL cholesterol and damage blood vessels, increasing the risk of heart disease. Quitting smoking can significantly improve cholesterol levels and overall cardiovascular health.

- Adequate Sleep: Quality sleep plays a role in cholesterol metabolism. Getting 7-9 hours of quality sleep per night supports overall health, including cholesterol levels.

- Weight Management: Maintaining a healthy weight through a balanced diet and regular exercise positively impacts cholesterol levels.

The Importance:

Lifestyle changes are fundamental in managing cholesterol levels because they address multiple aspects of heart health:

- Comprehensive Impact: Exercise, stress management, and lifestyle adjustments contribute to a comprehensive approach in managing cholesterol, impacting both LDL and HDL levels, triglycerides, and overall cardiovascular health.

- Sustainable Benefits: Unlike medications, lifestyle changes offer sustainable and long-term benefits, promoting overall health and reducing the risk of chronic diseases beyond just managing cholesterol.

- Synergistic Effects: When combined with dietary modifications, these lifestyle changes amplify the positive effects on cholesterol levels and overall heart health.

Adopting a holistic approach that includes regular physical activity, stress management techniques, and positive lifestyle adjustments not only aids in managing cholesterol but also fosters a healthier and more balanced life, reducing the risk of cardiovascular diseases and promoting overall well-being.

Chapter Six

Medications and Other Interventions

Certainly, medications and other interventions are sometimes necessary to manage cholesterol effectively, especially when lifestyle changes alone aren't sufficient or in cases where there's a higher risk of cardiovascular disease. Here are some interventions commonly used:

1. **Statins**:

- **Mechanism:** Statins are commonly prescribed medications that work by blocking an enzyme in the liver responsible for producing cholesterol. They primarily lower LDL cholesterol levels.

-Benefits: Statins not only reduce LDL cholesterol but also have been shown to lower the risk of heart attacks, strokes, and other cardiovascular events.

- Considerations: Side effects such as muscle pain or liver abnormalities can occur. Regular monitoring by a healthcare provider is essential when taking statins.

2. **Other Medications:**

- Ezetimibe: This medication lowers LDL cholesterol by blocking cholesterol absorption in the intestine.

-PCSK9 Inhibitors: These newer medications lower LDL cholesterol levels by increasing the liver's ability to remove LDL cholesterol from the blood. They are typically reserved for individuals with very high LDL cholesterol levels or those with familial hypercholesterolemia.

3. **Bile Acid Sequestrants:**

- Mechanism: These medications bind to bile acids in the intestines, helping to remove cholesterol from the body.

- Use: They can lower LDL cholesterol levels but may have gastrointestinal side effects.

4. Lifestyle Modification Support:

- Nutritional Counseling: Working with a registered dietitian can provide personalized dietary recommendations to manage cholesterol levels effectively.

- Exercise Programs: Structured exercise programs or guidance from a fitness professional can help individuals adopt and maintain regular physical activity.

5. Regular Monitoring:

- Lipid Profile Tests: Healthcare providers regularly monitor cholesterol levels to assess the effectiveness of interventions and make necessary adjustments to medications or lifestyle recommendations.

6. **Intervention in High-Risk Cases:**

- Familial Hypercholesterolemia: In cases of genetic conditions like familial hypercholesterolemia, where cholesterol levels are exceptionally high and lifestyle changes alone may not suffice, medications are often necessary from an early age.

- Post-Cardiovascular Events: After a heart attack or stroke, medications might be necessary to aggressively manage cholesterol levels and reduce the risk of subsequent events.

Medications and interventions are tailored to individual needs and risks. Healthcare providers assess an individual's overall health, cholesterol levels, risk factors, and potential side effects when recommending medications or interventions to manage cholesterol. These interventions are often complemented by lifestyle modifications to achieve optimal cholesterol management and reduce the risk of cardiovascular diseases. Regular discussions with a healthcare provider help determine the most suitable approach for managing cholesterol effectively.

Detailing pharmaceutical interventions like statins and their role in managing cholesterol.

Statins are a class of medications widely used to manage cholesterol levels, primarily targeting LDL (low-density lipoprotein) cholesterol. Here's an in-depth look at statins and their role in cholesterol management:

1. **Mechanism of Action:**

   - Inhibition of Cholesterol Production: Statins work by inhibiting an enzyme in the liver called HMG-CoA reductase, which is involved in producing cholesterol.

2. Effect on Cholesterol Levels:

- Lowering LDL Cholesterol: Statins are most effective in lowering LDL cholesterol levels, often referred to as "bad" cholesterol. They can reduce LDL cholesterol by 20% to 60%, depending on the specific statin, dosage, and individual response.

- Modest Effects on Triglycerides and HDL: While primarily targeting LDL cholesterol, statins might also modestly lower triglycerides and slightly increase HDL (high-density lipoprotein) cholesterol levels.

3. Benefits Beyond Cholesterol Lowering:

- Reducing Cardiovascular Risk: Statins have shown significant benefits in reducing the risk of heart attacks, strokes, and other cardiovascular events, especially in individuals at higher risk due to existing heart disease, diabetes, or other risk factors.

- Anti-inflammatory Effects: Some research suggests that statins might have anti-inflammatory properties beyond their cholesterol-lowering effects, contributing to their cardiovascular benefits.

4. Types of Statins:

- Common Statins: Examples include atorvastatin (Lipitor), simvastatin (Zocor), rosuvastatin (Crestor), lovastatin (Mevacor), and others. Each statin may have slightly different effects and dosages.

5. Considerations and Side Effects:

- Side Effects: Common side effects may include muscle aches or weakness, digestive issues, or liver abnormalities. Serious side effects are rare but might include muscle breakdown (rhabdomyolysis) or liver problems.

- Drug Interactions: Statins might interact with other medications, so it's essential to inform healthcare providers about all medications being taken to avoid potential interactions.

6. Individualized Treatment:

- Tailored Approach: The choice of statin, dosage, and duration of treatment is often individualized based on an individual's cholesterol levels, cardiovascular risk factors, medical history, and potential side effects.

7. Regular Monitoring:

- Lipid Profile Tests: Healthcare providers regularly monitor cholesterol levels and liver function tests to assess the effectiveness and safety of statin therapy.

Statins are considered a cornerstone in managing high cholesterol, especially for individuals at increased risk of cardiovascular diseases.

They play a crucial role in reducing LDL cholesterol levels and mitigating the risk of heart attacks, strokes, and other cardiovascular events. However, their use and dosage should be carefully monitored and personalized to balance benefits and potential side effects. Regular communication with a healthcare provider is essential when considering or using statin therapy for cholesterol management.

Discussing when medications might be necessary and their potential side effects.

Medications, particularly cholesterol-lowering drugs like statins, may be necessary in several scenarios:

1. **High Cholesterol Levels Persist Despite Lifestyle Changes:**

   - When healthy lifestyle modifications (diet, exercise, weight management) fail to sufficiently lower cholesterol levels, medications might be prescribed to help reach target levels.

2. **Presence of High Cardiovascular Risk:**

- Individuals with existing heart disease, diabetes, familial hypercholesterolemia, or multiple cardiovascular risk factors might require medications to aggressively manage cholesterol levels and reduce the risk of heart attacks, strokes, or other cardiovascular events.

3. Post-Cardiovascular Event Management:

- After experiencing a heart attack, stroke, or other cardiovascular events, medications are often prescribed to lower the risk of subsequent incidents.

4. Specific Medical Conditions:

- Certain medical conditions, genetic predispositions (like familial hypercholesterolemia), or liver diseases might necessitate medications to manage cholesterol levels.

Potential side effects of cholesterol-lowering medications, particularly statins, include:

1. **Muscle Pain or Weakness:**

- Some individuals may experience muscle-related symptoms, such as muscle pain, tenderness, or weakness, known as statin-associated myopathy. In rare cases, this can progress to severe muscle breakdown (rhabdomyolysis).

2. **Digestive Issues:**

- Statins can occasionally cause digestive problems like nausea, constipation, diarrhea, or abdominal pain.

3. **Liver Abnormalities:**

- In some cases, statins might lead to changes in liver enzyme levels. Regular monitoring of liver function tests is usually recommended.

4. Other Rare Side Effects:

- Rare side effects might include memory loss, confusion, or an increased risk of diabetes. However, the absolute risk of these side effects is generally low.

It's crucial to discuss the benefits and potential side effects of cholesterol-lowering medications with a healthcare provider. Healthcare professionals consider an individual's overall health, risk factors, potential drug interactions, and personal preferences when determining the necessity for medications and selecting the most suitable option.

In many cases, the benefits of reducing cardiovascular risk through cholesterol management outweigh the potential risks of medication side effects. However, open communication with healthcare providers and regular monitoring help in balancing the benefits and risks while ensuring optimal cholesterol management.

Chapter Seven:

Empowering Your Journey

Embarking on a journey to manage cholesterol and promote heart health is a significant step towards a healthier and more vibrant life. Here's how to empower your journey:

1. Education and Awareness:

   - **Knowledge is Key: Educate yourself about** cholesterol, its impact on health, and the role of lifestyle in managing it. Understanding empowers informed decisions.

2. Partnering with Healthcare Providers:

   - Open Communication: Build a collaborative relationship with healthcare professionals. Discuss concerns, goals, and treatment options openly. Ask questions and seek guidance to tailor a plan that suits your needs.

3. Setting Realistic Goals:

- Small Steps, Big Impact: Start with achievable lifestyle changes. Set realistic goals for diet, exercise, and stress management. Celebrate milestones, no matter how small.

4. Healthy Eating Habits:

- Focus on Nourishment:Embrace a diet rich in whole, nutrient-dense foods. Gradually reduce processed foods and unhealthy fats.

5. Regular Physical Activity:

- Make It Enjoyable: Find activities you love to maintain consistency. Aim for regular exercise sessions, even short ones. Consistency matters more than intensity.

6. Stress Management:

- Mindfulness and Relaxation: Incorporate stress-relieving practices into your daily routine. Explore meditation, yoga, deep breathing exercises, or hobbies that bring joy.

7. **Medication Compliance and Monitoring:**

- Stay Informed: If medications are prescribed, understand their purpose, benefits, and potential side effects. Adhere to prescribed regimens and attend regular check-ups for monitoring.

8. **Support Systems:**

- Community and Support: Engage with family, friends, or support groups.

9. **Celebrate Progress:**

- Acknowledge Achievements: Celebrate successes, whether it's making healthier food choices, increasing physical activity, or reaching cholesterol targets. Positive reinforcement boosts motivation.

10. **Adapt and Persist:**

- Flexibility and Perseverance: Embrace changes as part of a lifelong journey. Be adaptable and resilient. If setbacks occur, learn from them and keep moving forward.

11. Self-compassion:

- Kindness to Yourself: Be gentle and patient with yourself. Each step you take towards better heart health matters.

Empowering your journey involves a commitment to self-care, learning, and gradual but consistent changes. Your dedication to managing cholesterol and nurturing heart health is a remarkable investment in a healthier and more fulfilling life. Every effort you make brings you closer to a stronger, healthier heart and a brighter future.

Offering tips for maintaining motivation and sustaining healthy habits.

Absolutely! Maintaining motivation and sustaining healthy habits can be challenging but achievable. Here are tips to keep you motivated along your health journey:

1. Set Clear and Realistic Goals:

- Specific and Achievable: Define clear, realistic, and measurable goals. Break them into smaller milestones to track progress and celebrate achievements along the way.

2. Create a Supportive Environment:

- Surround Yourself: Engage with supportive friends, family, or communities sharing similar health goals. Their encouragement and shared experiences can boost motivation.

3. **Find Enjoyment in Activities:**

- Variety and Fun: Explore various physical activities until you find what you genuinely enjoy.

4. **Plan and Schedule:**

- Consistency Matters: Set a schedule for exercise, meal planning, and stress-relieving activities. Making them part of your routine helps maintain consistency.

5. **Focus on Progress, Not Perfection:**

- Celebrate Small Wins: Acknowledge and celebrate every positive step, no matter how small. Recognize progress as motivation to keep going.

6. **Mindful Eating and Moderation:**

- Balanced Choices: Practice mindful eating, savoring each bite. Aim for moderation rather than strict deprivation. Allow occasional treats without guilt.

7. **Track and Monitor Progress:**

- Keep Records: Use journals, apps, or tracking tools to monitor your food intake, exercise routine, or mood. Seeing improvements motivates continued efforts.

8. **Positive Self-talk and Mindset:**

- Encouraging Language: Replace negative self-talk with positive affirmations. Focus on what you've accomplished and believe in your ability to reach your goals.

9. **Adaptability and Flexibility:**

- Expect Changes: Embrace flexibility in your plan. Life brings surprises, so adapt and find ways to stay on track despite unexpected challenges.

10. Reward Yourself:

- Incentivize Progress: Set rewards for reaching milestones. These rewards serve as motivators and reinforce positive habits.

11. **Visualize Your Success:**

- Imagery and Vision: Create a mental image of your goals. Visualizing your success can fuel motivation and drive your efforts forward.

12. **Seek Inspiration:**

- Learn and Grow: Read success stories, follow inspirational figures, or educate yourself on health topics to stay motivated and gain new insights.

Remember, maintaining motivation is an ongoing process. There might be times when motivation dips, but by incorporating these strategies and staying committed to your health journey, you'll cultivate the resilience needed to sustain healthy habits over time. Celebrate your progress, stay focused on your goals, and be kind to yourself throughout the journey. Every step counts!

Addressing common challenges individuals face when managing cholesterol.

Certainly, managing cholesterol comes with its share of challenges. Here are some common hurdles individuals may encounter and strategies to overcome them:

1. **Dietary Challenges:**

- Unhealthy Food Temptations: Resisting unhealthy food choices, especially in social settings or when cravings strike, can be challenging.

- Strategy: Plan ahead by having healthy snacks available, practice mindful eating, and focus on the long-term benefits of a healthy diet.

2. **Exercise Obstacles:**

- Time Constraints: Finding time for regular exercise amid a busy schedule can be tough.

- Strategy: Incorporate short bursts of activity throughout the day, prioritize exercise by scheduling it, and choose activities that can be integrated into daily routines.

3. **Medication Adherence:**

- Forgetting Medications: Remembering to take medications regularly can be an issue for some individuals.

- Strategy: Use reminders such as alarms, pill organizers, or smartphone apps to stay on track with medications.

4. **Lack of Support:**

- Limited Support System: Not having a supportive environment or people around can make the journey more challenging.

- Strategy: Seek support from online communities, join local groups, or communicate your goals with friends and family to build a supportive network.

5.Financial Constraints:

- Cost of Healthier Options: Affordability of healthier food choices or gym memberships might be a concern.

- Strategy: Look for budget-friendly alternatives, explore local resources, use outdoor spaces for exercise, and plan meals that make the most of affordable, nutritious ingredients.

6. Medical Conditions and Side Effects:

- Managing Side Effects: Dealing with side effects from medications or health conditions can impact adherence to treatment.

- Strategy: Communicate openly with healthcare providers about any concerns or side effects. Explore alternative medications or lifestyle adjustments that might be more manageable.

7. **Plateauing Progress:**

- Lack of Visible Results: Plateauing in progress despite efforts can be disheartening.

- Strategy: Focus on non-scale victories, like improved energy levels, better sleep, or enhanced mood. Remember that small changes contribute to long-term health.

Addressing these challenges might require a combination of strategies, support systems, and a patient, persistent approach. Developing resilience and staying committed to your health goals will help overcome these obstacles and maintain progress towards managing cholesterol effectively.

Conclusion

As you journey toward better heart health and manage your cholesterol, remember this: every choice, every step, and every effort counts. Embrace the small victories, stay resilient through challenges, and celebrate your progress along the way. Your commitment to a healthier lifestyle isn't just about managing cholesterol; it's about empowering yourself to live a vibrant, fulfilling life. So, keep moving forward, stay focused on your goals, and cherish the incredible impact you're making on your heart and overall well-being. Here's to a heart-healthy, empowered you!